Melissa Connor

Camel milk the Delicious Liquid Gold

Contents

Introduction

From the deserts, a new kind of milk emerged. We call this popular and delicious fellow "camel's milk"

Although camel milk differs in composition from cow milk, the exact ratios of its constituent elements can vary greatly depending on a variety of factors such as the camel's breed, environment, diet, and milking technique. Yogurt and ice cream are possible end products, but making butter or cheese from it is more of a challenge.

The camel's milk has many perpetuated health benefits. Keep reading to find out more.

Chapter 1

What is Camel milk and what does it taste like?

Camel milk as the name suggests is milk gotten from camels. It is very delicious and creamy, the milk of the American camel is similar to normal milk in taste but with a salty and sweet aftertaste that keeps you wanting more while camel milk from the middle east has a more smoky and nutty flavour, yummy..

Popular amongst the nomad and pastoral cultures. Over a millenia ago, herders may have survived solely on Camel milk over periods when grazing long distances in arid and

desert regions especially in the
Middle East and North Africa.

Camel milk Nutrients
- Vitamin A
- Vitamin C
- Vitamin E
- Vitamin B
- Vitamin D
- Calcium
- Kalium
- Potassium
- Magnesium
- Iron
- Copper
- Thiamine
- Riboflavin
- Phosphorus

Chapter 2

Camel milk Benefits

Immune system and antimicrobial activity

There are different immune protein molecules in camel milk that can fight off different microbes and act as protection. Immunoglobulins in milk can kill bacteria that cause diseases like tuberculosis. Also, it can protect the body from getting sick from bacteria and viruses. Lactoferrin, which is found in camel milk, can stop the growth of infectious microbes and is part of the immune system. Also, putting lactoperoxidase from milk out in the open could kill bacteria, especially gram-negative bacteria. Some researchers have found that camel milk helps people with tuberculosis, especially those who are resistant to multiple drugs. In a study about camel milk that had been pasteurized, the results showed that camel milk has antimicrobial activity against pathogens that come from food. Also, it was seen that pasteurization has no effect on the ability to kill bacteria. Many studies have shown that camel milk kills bacteria and other germs.

Diabetes with camel milk

Camel milk is easy to spot because it is low in fat and cholesterol and is full of vitamins and minerals. It is also a good source of insulin. It has been talked about how camel milk can help people with diabetes. It was found that there was about 32 U/ml of insulin in camel milk.

It has been reported that camel milk can be used to treat type 2 diabetes because it has a lot of insulin in it. So, camel milk can be used along with insulin to treat type 2 diabetes. This can help reduce the amount of insulin needed, especially if it is safe and effective at controlling diabetes over the long term.

Camel milk could be safe and effective in long-term glycemic control and reducing the need for insulin doses in people with type I diabetes.

The regenerative properties of camel milk are remarkable.
Many of the chemicals used in expensive cosmetics and medical treatments may be found in camel milk. Alpha-hydroxy acids are one example of such a component; they help smooth fine lines and wrinkles, exfoliate dead skin, and balance out skin tone. Also, it doesn't irritate your skin. In other words, it's a fantastic natural alternative for people who have extremely sensitive skin and can't use over-the-counter or prescription medications.

Anti-aging ingredients like collagen, elastin, and lanolin are found in camel milk as well, allowing it to effectively seal in moisture while also bolstering the skin's firmness, elasticity, and strength. Want to restore your hair's natural luster and suppleness? Try drinking some camel's milk. It's no surprise that Cleopatra relied on this for flawless hair and skin.

One of the most promising therapies for behavioral disorders is camel milk.

In recent years, it has come to light that drinking camel milk might help alleviate some of the symptoms of neurodegenerative disorders including Parkinson's disease,

Alzheimer's disease, and others. Camel milk's antioxidant qualities are likely responsible for the observed enhancements.

Camel milk has anti inflammatory properties

Camel milk's anti-inflammatory properties make it useful for treating a variety of inflammatory disorders, including bronchitis and arthritis.

Milk-allergic people can drink camel milk safely.

One possible option that is less risky is camel milk, if you have one. Possible explanation: camel milk has a kind of protein that doesn't create an allergic reaction in the body, unlike other dairy products. There are additional food allergies that camel milk can assist with as well.

Autistic Behavior and Camel Milk

Communication and social interaction difficulties are hallmarks of autism, a disorder of neurodevelopment that persists throughout a person's life. Due to its high antioxidant content in the form of vitamins A, C, and E, as well as other minerals like Mg and Zn, camel milk has been proven to be effective in treating autistic people by lowering their oxidative stress rate. Additionally, these minerals have been shown to include antibodies of the same size as immunological antibodies in people, which is functioning to promote autistic behavior by stimulating glutathione production. Some neurological disorders, such as autism, have been linked to oxidative stress. Camel milk has recently been found to have a significant therapeutic effect on autistic symptoms.

Camel milk and the Crohn syndrome

Crohn syndrome is an inflammatory disorder that can affect any part of the body, from the mouth to the anus. It can make you lose weight, have stomach pain, throw up, or have diarrhea or vomiting. It could also cause more health problems, like eye inflammation, tiredness, trouble focusing, skin rashes, and arthritis. Most of the time, this disease is caused by things in the environment, in the immune system, or in microbes. In particular, the microorganism mycobacterium avium-subspecies causes paratuberculosis in cow milk, which can't be stopped by heating. People have used and suggested camel milk as a way to treat Crohn diseases. It has been said that camel milk can be used to treat this bacterium because it comes from the same family as tuberculosis.

Other benefits of camel milk include

It is a better alternative for those with high cholesterol.

It helps with food allergies

It is a great option for those that are lactose intolerant.

It is great for boosting your immunity while having a chilled or hot glass of delicious creamy milk.

GABA is an amino acid found in abundance in camel milk. Because of this, you may find that your infant sleeps better after a feeding of camel milk formula.

Chapter 3

Some Camel milk recipes

Camel milk baby formula
Ingredients
½ tsp Cod liver oil, unflavored

¼ tsp Acerola, powder

2 teaspoons of nutrition yeast

¼ tsp Butter oil, unflavored

2 tsp Coconut oil, virgin

1 tsp extra-virgin olive oil, preferably organic

1 teaspoon of sunflower oil

2 cups Camel milk, raw or camel milk kefir

¼ cup liquid whey

4 tablespoons Fresh or pasteurized cream

2 tsp Gelatin, unflavored
1 ⅞ cup filtered water
¼ tsp Powder made from
Bifidobacterium infantis
4 Tbl lactose

Instructions
=>Fill a Pyrex measuring cup that
holds 2 cups with filtered water and
take out 2 tablespoons. This will give
you 1 ⅞ cups of water.

=>About half of the water goes into a
pan, and the burner is set to medium.

=>Add the gelatin and lactose and let
them dissolve while you stir them
every now and then.

=>When the gelatin and lactose are dissolved, take the pan off the heat and add the rest of the water to cool it down.

=>Mix in the butter oil and coconut oil until they are melted.

=>Mix the rest of the ingredients together in a glass blender.

=>Blend for about 3 seconds after adding the water mixture.

=>Put formula in a glass baby bottle or jar and put it in the fridge.

=>Warm up the glass bottle in a pan of hot water or a bottle warmer before giving it to the baby. NEVER heat baby bottles in a microwave!

Important Notes on the Recipe

Don't use powdered whey from the store, as it has been changed in some way. If you use whey from making cheese, the formula will turn sour.

Don't substitute pasteurized or powdered milk. These are heavily processed, denatured foods that can cause allergies.

Don't use ultra pasteurized (UHT) cream. It causes a lot of allergies. Either raw or pasteurized cream is fine.

If you don't have enough gelatin, you can use collagen powder instead.

For this recipe, you should only use organic, cold-pressed, unrefined, low-oleic sunflower oil.

Gelatin is to blame if the formula gets a little thicker after being in the fridge for a while. When you warm it up for your baby's next bottle, it will become liquid again.

Camel's drool
Ingredients
Eggs
Cooked condensed milk
Grated biscuit for garnish

Directions

It's time to separate the egg whites from the yolks. The egg whites should be beaten until stiff and placed aside.

Blend the egg yolks and sweetened condensed milk together in a bowl using a wire whisk. The beaten egg whites should then be folded in carefully using a spatula.

Divide the dessert among separate glass dishes and chill for at least four hours.

Take dessert out of the fridge and sprinkle shredded biscuits on top before serving.

Camel milk cake tart

Ingredients

15 Kg camel milk

1500 gms sugar

15 ml vinegar

250 gms butter

500 gms brown sugar

75 gms refined flour

2 eggs

Directions

1. Get a big bowl.

2.Mix together all of the dry and wet ingredients to make dough.

3.Roll the dough out gently and put it in the mold to give it a shape.

4.Bake at 180'c for 20 minutes.

5.Let the tart cool all the way down.

6. Garnish (optional)

Camel milk pancakes
Ingredients
400 grams of wheat berries
Camel milk, half a liter
Fine Sugar, 30 Grams
sugar, vanilla, 1 teaspoon
4 eggs
Sunflower oil, to taste
Butter

Preparation
Use a hand mixer or a whisk to combine the flour, sugar, vanilla sugar, eggs, camel milk, and a pinch of sunflower oil in a bowl.

Be cautious to preheat your baking pan because the oil in the batter will reduce the amount of fat you use in the final product. A little butter on a hot pan is all you need to begin cooking. Cover the pancake stack with a lid or a plate to keep it warm during baking.

Shubat
Ingredients
10.0 grams of dry milk powder
Camel milk, 500 grams
Kefir cereal on demand

Instructions
Add one cup of camel milk powder to a saucepan.
Camel milk should be heated to a temperature of 92 degrees Fahrenheit, so place the pot on high heat (or thereabouts).

Mix in the kefir grains.

Because of the lack of significant thickening, it is hard to identify when the milk is ready to be strained. Once a thin layer of liquid has formed at the bottom of the bowl and the milk has begun to separate from the rest of the ingredients, you may proceed to the next stage.

When the mixture is the right temperature and consistency, remove it from the heat and transfer it to a bowl. Stir the filtered Shubat and drink it.

Put a cover on the saucepan and pour the contents into glass containers.

After filling the jars, let the liquid sit undisturbed for 18 to 24 hours in a cool, dry area (like a closet).
Bottoms up!

Camel milk frittata
Ingredients
6 eggs
300ml of camel milk
1 large sweet potato
3 large tomatoes
Fresh basil and spinach, about 2 handfuls
⅓ cup of dried Parmesan
1 cup shredded cheese (cheddar is a good option)
½ tsp pepper
1 pinch of salt
1 tablespoon of dry chives

Olive oil spray

Instructions

=>Turn the oven on for 20 minutes at 200C.

=>Eggs, camel milk, pepper, salt, and parmesan cheese should be mixed together until they have the consistency of custard.

=>Before cutting the sweet potato into thin slices, peel it and partially cook it.

=>Cut three tomatoes into thin slices.

=>Use olive oil spray to coat a baking dish well.

=>Sweet potatoes are used to line the dish. After that, put a layer of tomatoes on top. Add some dried chives. Add a layer of spinach, then another layer of tomatoes and dried chives. Then put a layer of basil on top.

=>Pour the "custard," which is a mixture of egg and camel milk, over the stack of vegetables.

=>Grate a cup of cheese and sprinkle it all over the dish.

=>Bake in an oven that has already been heated until the "custard" has hardened and the cheese has turned brown.

Camel milk chocolate fondue

Ingredients

1¼ cups or 280 grams of bittersweet or semisweet chocolate chips (milk or dark)

½ to ¾ cup of camel milk

2 tbsp butter

1 tsp vanilla extract

Instructions

=>Mix chocolate, camel milk, and butter in a bowl or pan that can take heat.

=>Put the bowl on top of a pot of water that is slowly boiling, and melt it slowly. You can also melt it in a microwave for two minutes on medium power. Mix until it's smooth. If the mix is too thick or lumpy, add more camel milk

=>Stir in vanilla extract.

=>Fondue can be eaten right away or put aside and heated up again later.

=>Prepare dipping ingredients: marshmallows, banana pieces, apple pieces, pineapple chunks, strawberries, bite-sized pieces of sponge cake.

Conclusion

The amazing thing about this delicious milk is that it can replace the usual milk in a lot of recipes. So whether you have a sweet tooth or you are diabetic, there is a camel milk recipe for you.

Knowing the wonders the white gold is capable of, are you willing to add it to your diet now? Even if you don't use it cook, what about drinking a glass a day or every other day depending on your finances?

I personally recommend this camel milk and I hope you have fun trying

out the various recipes listed in the
book.

Finally, we have come to the end of
this book, it was a very short one, i
know. I hope you enjoyed it. Please
leave a review if you did. Thank you

www.ingramcontent.com/pod-product-compliance
Lightning Source LLC
Chambersburg PA
CBHW071217260726
48653CB00041B/982